EATING GUIDE FOR THE LOW OXALATE DIET

Prevent Kidney Stones and Hyperoxaluria, Manage Vulvodynia, Maintain Renal Health, Reduce Gastrointestinal Discomfort, and Improve Overall Well-being

Audrey McAllister, MD

Copyright Page

laws and regulations. By accessing or using any part of this work, individuals agree to comply with the terms and conditions set forth by the publisher regarding copyright protection and usage rights.

Table of Contents

SECTION I: UNDERSTANDING OXALATES

Oxalates are naturally occurring compounds that are found in a wide variety of plant foods. They are organic acids that are produced by plants as a defense mechanism against herbivores. Oxalates have a unique structure, consisting of a carbon atom bonded to four oxygen atoms. The presence of oxalates in plants is essential for their survival, as they help to prevent damage from insects and other pests.

The chemical structure of oxalates makes them highly reactive, and they have the ability to bind with minerals such as calcium and form insoluble crystals. These oxalate crystals can accumulate in various tissues and organs of the body, leading to the formation of kidney stones or other health problems. It is important to note that not all oxalates are harmful, and some are even beneficial for human health. However, excessive consumption of oxalate-rich foods can cause issues for certain individuals, particularly those who are susceptible to kidney stone formation.

In human health and nutrition, oxalates play a complex role. On one hand, they can interfere with the absorption of certain minerals, such as calcium and iron, by binding to them and forming insoluble complexes. Consequently, this can lead to mineral deficiencies, especially in individuals who have a diet high in oxalates and low in minerals. On the other hand, oxalates have been shown to have antioxidant properties and may offer some health benefits, including the prevention of oxidative stress and inflammation.

However, it is worth noting that the health effects of oxalates can vary greatly depending on an individual's overall diet, health status, and genetic factors. While some people can tolerate moderate amounts of oxalates without any issues, others may be more sensitive and experience adverse effects. It is essential to strike a balance and consume a varied diet that includes a mix of oxalate-containing foods and other nutrient-rich sources to ensure optimal health and nutrition.

How are we exposed to oxalic acid?

We are exposed to oxalic acid through various sources. Here are some common ways we can come into contact with oxalic acid:

• **Dietary Sources:** Many plant-based foods naturally contain oxalic acid; when we consume these foods, we expose ourselves to oxalic acid.

• **Cooking and Food Preparation**: Cooking methods like boiling, steaming, and blanching vegetables can help reduce oxalic acid content versus eating foods high in oxalic acid raw.

- **Oxalate Supplements:** Some supplements that promote kidney health or manage specific medical conditions may contain oxalic acid or oxalate salts.

- **Occupational Exposure:** Some industries, such as metal cleaning and polishing, use oxalic acid for various purposes. Workers in these industries may come into contact with oxalic acid through direct contact or inhalation.

- **Household Products:** Household cleaning products, including rust removers, wood bleachers, or cleaning agents, sometimes contain oxalic acid.

- **Fungal infections or Mold Exposure:** Ongoing research suggests that fungal infections or colonization or mold exposure may lead to increased oxalic acid production in the body.

Even though oxalic acid is naturally occurring and generally safe in moderate amounts, excessive or prolonged exposure to high levels of oxalic acid can be harmful.

Testing for Oxalates

Testing for oxalates is done through a urine test, but it may not accurately reflect the overall oxalate burden in the body. Here's why:

• Timing and variability: Oxalate levels in urine can vary throughout the day and from day to day.

• Dietary influence: Recent intake of high-oxalate foods can affect urine oxalate levels.

• Absorption and excretion: Factors like gut health and metabolism impact how oxalates are absorbed and utilized.

• Tissue deposition: Urine oxalate levels may not reflect oxalate accumulation in tissues.

Your healthcare provider must interpret your oxalate test results in the context of your symptoms, medical history, and overall health so that you can receive personalized guidance and treatment options.

Treatment for Elevated Oxalate Levels

The treatment for elevated oxalate levels depends on the underlying cause and the specific health condition. Here are some general approaches to consider:

• **Dietary Modifications:** Adjusting your diet to reduce oxalate intake can help manage elevated oxalate levels. This should be done by slowly reducing high-oxalate foods to avoid oxalate dumping and worsening of symptoms.

• **Calcium and Vitamin B6 Supplementation**: When taken with meals, calcium supplements or calcium-rich foods can bind to the digestive tract's oxalates and reduce their absorption. Vitamin B6 may also be recommended, as it plays a role in oxalate metabolism.

• **Gut Health Optimization:** Supporting a healthy gut microbiome through a balanced diet, probiotics, and prebiotic-rich foods can enhance oxalate metabolism and reduce oxalate-related issues.

• **Medications:** If you have specific underlying medical conditions that cause elevated oxalate levels, your doctor may prescribe medications to reduce oxalate production or enhance oxalate breakdown.

Sources of Oxalates in Foods

Oxalates are found in a wide range of foods, both plant-based and animal-based. Some of the primary sources of oxalates include spinach, rhubarb, beet greens, Swiss chard, kale, cocoa powder, nuts, seeds, and certain types of berries. It is important to note that cooking or processing foods can sometimes reduce the oxalate content, making them more tolerable for individuals who are sensitive to oxalates. However, it is still advisable to consume oxalate-rich foods in moderation and in conjunction with other nutrient-dense foods to minimize potential health risks.

Leafy greens, legumes, and other foods high in oxalates are rich in beneficial nutrients. However, because oxalates bind to calcium as they leave the body, they can increase the risk of kidney stones in some people.

High-Oxalate Foods

High-oxalate foods include:

1. Spinach

Leafy greens like spinach contain many vitamins and minerals, but they're also high in oxalates. A half-cup of cooked spinach contains 755 milligrams.

2. Soy products

Products made from soybeans are excellent sources of protein and other nutrients, especially for people on a plant-based diet. However, they are also high in oxalates. A 3-ounce serving of firm tofu has 235 milligrams, while 1 cup of soy milk or yogurt can have up to 336 milligrams per serving.

3. Almonds

Almonds are concentrated with a range of vitamins and minerals, yet they are also high in oxalates. One ounce of almonds, or about 22 nuts, contains 122 milligrams of oxalates.

4. Potatoes

A medium baked potato has 97 milligrams of oxalates per serving. Much of this content is in the potato's skin, which contains high levels of nutrients like fiber, vitamin C, and B vitamins.

5. Beets

Beets are an excellent source of nutrients like folate and manganese. Research shows their nitric oxide content helps lower your blood pressure. At 152 milligrams per cup, they're also one of the vegetables highest in oxalates.

6. Navy beans

Legumes are a great way to add protein, fiber, and other nutrients to any meal. However, if you're managing your oxalate levels, navy beans are on the high end with 76 milligrams per half-cup.

7. Raspberries

Many fruits contain some oxalates, like avocados, oranges, and grapefruit, but raspberries are considered a high-oxalate food with 48 milligrams per cup.

8. Dates

Dates are highly nutritious dried fruits often used as a sweetener in cooking and baking. Date consumption should be moderated, however, as they are high in sugar and concentrated with oxalates with one date containing 24 milligrams.

For individuals who are at a higher risk of kidney stone formation or have a history of kidney stones, it may be necessary to limit the consumption of foods high in oxalates. Additionally, it is crucial to stay well-hydrated and maintain a balanced diet to help reduce the risk of stone formation. Working with a healthcare professional or nutritionist can provide personalized guidance on managing oxalate intake and ensuring optimal nutrition while minimizing potential health risks.

Health Implications of High Oxalate Consumption

Oxalates are associated with various symptoms and conditions, particularly when levels are elevated or if you're sensitive to their effects. Some common symptoms and conditions associated with oxalates include:

• **Kidney Stones:** High levels of oxalates in the urine can contribute to the formation of kidney stones. These stones can cause severe pain, blood in the urine, and discomfort in the lower back or abdomen.

• **Urinary Tract Issues:** Oxalates can irritate the urinary tract and potentially contribute to urinary tract infections or inflammation.

• **Gastrointestinal Symptoms:** Some people may experience GI symptoms related to oxalate consumption, such as bloating, gas, abdominal pain, or changes in bowel movements.

• **Nutrient Deficiencies:** Oxalates can bind to minerals like calcium and magnesium, hindering their absorption. This can lead to deficiencies if dietary intake is not correctly balanced.

• **Vulvodynia:** In some cases, oxalates have been associated with vulvodynia, characterized by chronic pain, discomfort, or burning in the vulva area.

• **Joint and Muscle Pain:** People with specific metabolic disorders that affect oxalate metabolism commonly experience joint and muscle pain.

• **Hyperoxaluria:** This condition is characterized by excessive oxalate production or impaired oxalate metabolism, leading to elevated levels of oxalates in the body. This can increase the risk of kidney stones and other related complications.

Some people may be more sensitive to oxalates than others, and the severity and presence of symptoms may vary. If you suspect oxalate-related issues, talk with your healthcare provider, who can evaluate your symptoms, conduct appropriate tests, and provide personalized guidance and treatment options based on your situation.

The Connection between Oxalates and Gut Health

The connection between oxalates and gut health is an area of growing interest and research. Oxalates can interact with the gut in several ways, including:

• **Oxalate Metabolism:** Gut bacteria metabolize oxalates from food, breaking them down into harmless byproducts or converting them for absorption. Dysbiosis, an imbalance in gut bacteria, can disrupt this process, impacting how the body handles oxalates.

• **Oxalate Absorption:** A healthy gut usually results in poor oxalate absorption and excretion in stool. But changes in gut microbiota or intestinal health can enhance oxalate absorption, causing high levels.

• **Gut Irritation and Inflammation**: In some people, high levels of oxalates in the gut can contribute to gut irritation and inflammation, which can result in bloating, abdominal pain, diarrhea, or changes in bowel movements.

• **Impact on Nutrient Absorption:** Oxalates can bind to minerals like calcium, magnesium, and iron, forming insoluble compounds. This can interfere with the absorption of these essential minerals in the gut.

Some people may be more sensitive to oxalate-related gut issues, while others may tolerate them. Managing oxalate intake, promoting a healthy gut microbiota, and addressing any underlying gut issues are potential strategies for supporting gut health in relation to oxalates.

SECTION II: BENEFITS OF A LOW OXALATE DIET

Conditions that Benefit from a Low Oxalate Diet

Some research shows that increased oxalate intake may be linked to greater excretion of oxalate through the urine, which may contribute to the development of kidney stones.

However, increasing your intake of calcium may be an effective way to help protect against kidney stones. This approach provides an alternative to eliminating foods that are high in oxalate.

In fact, consuming more calcium can help decrease the absorption of oxalate in your body, which could prevent kidney stones from forming.

One 10-person study even found that consuming high amounts of oxalate did not increase the risk of developing calcium oxalate kidney stones when participants were meeting the daily recommended intake for calcium.

However, this study was small, and scientists need to do more research on the topic.

Recommendations suggest aiming for 1,000–1,200 mg of calcium per day, which you can find in foods like dairy products, leafy greens, sardines, and seeds.

Here are a few other ways to reduce the risk of calcium oxalate kidney stones:

• **Limit salt intake.** Studies show that consuming high amounts of salt may be linked to a higher risk of developing kidney stones.

• **Avoid vitamin C supplements.** Your body converts vitamin C into oxalate, so avoid using high-dose vitamin C supplements unless your healthcare provider recommends it.

• **Stay hydrated.** Increasing your fluid intake can increase urine output and reduce the risk of kidney stones.

Other benefits

Some people claim that oxalates may be associated with other health problems, including autism.

In fact, one small study found that children with autism had significantly higher levels of oxalate in their blood and urine compared with a control group.

However, there's no research suggesting that autism is caused by dietary oxalates or showing any potential benefit of a low oxalate diet for treating autism.

People have also used low oxalate diets to treat vulvodynia, a condition characterized by chronic pain of the vulva.

Studies show that dietary oxalate consumption is not associated with a higher risk of developing vulvodynia. However, following a low oxalate diet may help with pain management.

Foods necessary for Supporting Low Oxalate Diets

1. Kale and bok choy

If you're watching your intake of oxalates, kale and bok choy are nutrient-rich greens with just 2 milligrams and 1 milligram of oxalates per cup, respectively.

2. Cashews, peanuts, and walnuts

Compared to almonds, nuts like cashews, peanuts, and walnuts have slightly lower levels of oxalates at about 30 milligrams per ounce.

3. Pumpkin and sunflower seeds

One ounce of pumpkin and sunflower seeds contain less than 2 milligrams of oxalates. They're also a good source of vitamin E, magnesium, and protein.

4. Sweet potatoes

You can swap your baked potato for sweet potatoes, which are higher in most vitamins and minerals and only have 28 milligrams of oxalates per cup.

5. Broccoli

Broccoli is a delicious low-oxalate vegetable at just 2 milligrams per cup. It's also a good source of fiber and protein and contains many important nutrients and vitamins.

6. Kidney beans

Kidney beans are a good substitute for navy beans with only 15 milligrams per half-cup. They're also a rich source of protein and fiber.

7. Blueberries and blackberries

Mix other berries in with your raspberries to reduce your oxalate intake. Blueberries and blackberries have only 4 milligrams of oxalates per cup. They're also rich in antioxidants, which can help prevent diseases such as heart disease and cancer.

8. Dried figs

For a sweet fix that's lower in oxalates, try dried figs, which have one-fifth of the dates' content. They're also high in fiber, potassium, iron, and calcium.

Potential Health Benefits Beyond Oxalate Reduction

Successfully reducing high oxalate foods could reduce the formation of kidney stones.

May Reduce Risk of Developing Kidney Stones

The conclusion is that oxalates from your diet impact kidney stone formation. Though researchers are not sure of the extent, the risk is there. Therefore, reducing your intake of high-oxalate foods might help you avoid future kidney stones.

Other health benefits associated with this diet include improved digestive health, reduced inflammation, and better absorption of nutrients. This diet may also be beneficial for individuals with certain autoimmune conditions and chronic pain syndromes.

SECTION III: PLANNING A LOW OXALATE DIET

Guidelines and Recommendations for Reducing Oxalates

If you are at risk for the development of calcium oxalate kidney stones, the following is recommended in order to decrease oxalate levels.

Increase fluid intake

This may be the easiest and most effective way to avoid developing kidney stones.

Increasing your fluids helps thin out your urine and makes it tougher for chemicals to build up and form crystals. Consult your healthcare provider for the amount of fluids that are recommended for you.

Avoid eating too much protein

Too much protein can lead to calcium oxalate stones to form, according to the National Kidney Foundation.

Lessen salt (sodium) intake

A diet that is high in sodium can cause calcium to build up in your urine. Having too much calcium in your urine can potentially cause new stones to form.

Consume calcium-rich foods

Calcium is found in milk and dairy foods like cheese and yogurt. It's recommended to eat foods high in calcium over taking a supplement. Speak to a registered dietitian nutritionist to help find the best sources of calcium in your diet. Too much or too little calcium can lead to the formation of calcium oxalate kidney stones.

The National Kidney Foundation recommends consuming three servings of milk and dairy foods – one serving at each meal. However, a RDN will to look at your urine, blood tests and medical conditions before making a final recommendation that is customized to you and your needs. The following are calcium-rich foods that are recommended on a low-oxalate diet:

• Whole, reduced fat, low fat, and skim milk.

• Plain yogurt or with allowed fruit like cherry, peach, banana and mango.

• Soy, almond and rice beverages fortified with calcium.

• Sardines with soft bones.

• Plain soy-based yogurt or with allowed fruit cherry, peach, banana and mango.

• Cheese.

• Kefir.

• Lentils and beans.

Avoid vitamin C supplements

Too much vitamin C can lead to high oxalate levels in the urine, which can increase the risk of stone formation. Speak with your healthcare provider before taking a vitamin C supplement.

Consume less oxalate-rich foods

Although most oxalate-rich foods are nutrient-rich, the National Kidney Foundation recommends limiting how many oxalate-rich foods you eat daily. Foods with high oxalate levels that should be avoided include nuts, rhubarb, beets, chocolate soy milk, All Bran cereal, buckwheat flour, miso, tahini, sesame seeds, and Swiss chard.

Practical Tips for Grocery Shopping and Meal Planning

Meal planning and preparation are necessary components of successfully adopting a low-oxalate diet. The following strategies can help ensure your meals are balanced, varied, and aligned with your goals. With a clear plan, navigating the grocery store and making decisions in the kitchen can become manageable. Consider the following recommendations when planning meals and snacks:

Educate Yourself

Familiarize yourself with the oxalate content of different foods. Keep a list of high, moderate, and low-oxalate foods handy, and refer to it when planning your meals. This will help you make informed decisions and create a well-rounded low-oxalate diet. When eating foods that are moderate in oxalate content, limit your intake to no more than two servings a day.

Seek Variety

Aim for a diverse range of foods in your meals to ensure you receive a broad spectrum of nutrients. Eat low-oxalate vegetables, fruits, grains, pasta, and lean proteins to add variety to your diet while keeping oxalate levels in check. Eating the same foods each day can be boring and may lead to inadequate nutrient intake. Having a variety of foods available helps you stay on track and may make it easier to adhere to your diet.

Portion Control

Moderation is key, especially for foods with moderate oxalate content. Pay attention to portion sizes to help manage your overall oxalate intake. Remember, it's not just about eliminating high oxalate foods but also being mindful of how much moderate oxalate foods you consume.

Read Food Labels

When grocery shopping, read food labels carefully. Look for hidden sources of oxalates, such as packaged foods, sauces, and condiments. In addition, some food additives or preservatives may contain oxalates, so it's important to be aware of their presence in processed items. When it comes to making healthier choices, reading labels is vital.

Plan Ahead

Set aside dedicated time for meal planning and preparation. Create a weekly meal plan, make a shopping list, and batch cook when possible. Having low-oxalate meals and snacks readily available can help you stay on track and avoid making impulsive food choices. If you are having trouble coming up with ideas, many recipe-finder tools online can help you find delicious and nutritious low-oxalate recipes.

Sample Meal Plans and Recipes

Monday

Breakfast

Scrambled eggs with spinach and feta cheese, gluten-free toast, and a cup of black tea

Lunch

Grilled chicken breast with roasted sweet potato and green beans, and a glass of water

Dinner

Baked salmon with quinoa and steamed broccoli, and a cup of herbal tea

Snacks

Sliced apple with almond butter and a handful of unsalted mixed nuts

Tuesday

Breakfast

Greek yogurt with blueberries and chia seeds, and a cup of green tea

Lunch

Tuna salad with mixed greens, cherry tomatoes, and cucumber, and a glass of water

Dinner

Grilled sirloin steak with mashed sweet potato and sautéed kale, and a cup of herbal tea

Snacks

Carrot sticks with hummus and a small piece of dark chocolate

Wednesday

Breakfast

Oatmeal with sliced banana and walnuts, and a cup of black tea

Lunch

Roasted turkey breast with roasted butternut squash and Brussels sprouts, and a glass of water

Dinner

Stir-fried shrimp with brown rice and mixed vegetables, and a cup of herbal tea

Snacks

Celery sticks with cream cheese and a handful of dried apricots

Thursday

Breakfast

Smoothie bowl with mixed berries, almond milk, and granola, and a cup of green tea

Lunch

Grilled chicken breast with roasted zucchini and yellow squash, and a glass of water

Dinner

Baked cod with roasted asparagus and quinoa, and a cup of herbal tea

Snacks

Hard-boiled egg with cherry tomatoes and a small piece of cheese

Friday

Breakfast

Avocado toast with smoked salmon and a cup of black tea

Lunch

Mixed greens salad with grilled chicken, cherry tomatoes, and cucumber, and a glass of water

Dinner

Grilled pork chop with roasted sweet potato and green beans, and a cup of herbal tea

Snacks

Sliced pear with almond butter and a handful of roasted almonds

Saturday

Breakfast

Scrambled eggs with sautéed mushrooms and gluten-free toast, and a cup of green tea

Lunch

Grilled shrimp with mixed greens, cherry tomatoes, and cucumber, and a glass of water

Dinner

Baked chicken breast with roasted butternut squash and Brussels sprouts, and a cup of herbal tea

Snacks

Sliced cucumber with tzatziki sauce and a small piece of dark chocolate

Sunday

Breakfast

Smoothie with mixed berries, spinach, and almond milk, and a cup of black tea

Lunch

Grilled salmon with roasted zucchini and yellow squash, and a glass of water

Dinner

Stir-fried beef with brown rice and mixed vegetables, and a cup of herbal tea

Snacks

Sliced apple with peanut butter and a handful of unsalted mixed nuts

SECTION IV: LOW OXALATE DIET RECIPES

BREAKFAST RECIPES FOR LOW OXALATE DIET

2 Ingredient English Muffin Recipe

INGREDIENTS

- 2 teaspoon butter

- 1½ cups mozzarella cheese shredded

- 2 large eggs

INSTRUCTIONS

1. Preheat the oven to 350 °F (175°C). Grease a 6-cup muffin pan with butter.

2. Combine cheese and eggs together in a large mixing bowl.

3. Divide the batter and fill each muffin space evenly.

4. Bake for 20 minutes, until tops are golden brown.

5. Run a knife around the edges to loosen each muffin. Remove from the pan and cool on a wire rack.

Hot Keto Cereal (Low-Carb Oatmeal)

INGREDIENTS

- ½ cup coconut flour

- ¼ cup flax seed

- ¼ cup chia seed

- 3 cups water

- ¼ cup Keto sugar substitute

- 1 teaspoon ground cinnamon

- 1 teaspoon vanilla extract

- ¼ teaspoon salt

- 4 whole eggs whisked

- 4 tablespoons coconut cream

Optional Add-ins:

- ¼ cup berries

- 1 tablespoon almond butter

- 1 tablespoon unsweetened shredded coconut

- 1 tablespoon hemp seeds

- 1 tablespoon cacao nibs

INSTRUCTIONS

1. Combine coconut flour, flax, and chia with the water in a small saucepan over medium heat. Cook for about 5 minutes, as it comes to a simmer.

2. Mix sweeter, cinnamon, vanilla, and salt in a small bowl. Add to the pot and stir to combine.

3. Reduce heat to low. Stir in the whisked eggs and continue cooking until cereal has thickened, approximately 5 minutes.

4. Serve warm with cream on top. Divide optional add-ins equally between all servings.

Carnivore Pancakes Recipe with 2-Ingredients

INGREDIENTS

• 4 ounces cream cheese

• 4 large eggs

• 1 teaspoon butter for frying

Optional Add-ins

• ¼ teaspoon salt

• 1 tablespoon Keto sugar substitute

• ½ tablespoon butter for serving

• ½ cup whipped cream for serving

• 1 tablespoon honey or maple, for serving, if not keto

INSTRUCTIONS

1. Blend the cream cheese and eggs in a blender.

2. Heat the butter in a skillet over medium heat.

3. Scoop the batter with a 1 tablespoon a measuring spoon and pour onto the pan.

4. Cook, until the edges separate from the pan and you can easily slip a spatula under the pancake to flip it over.

5. Flip and cook the second side until it turns golden brown.

6. Remove from heat and set aside. Then, continue cooking all the batter until done.

2-Ingredient Keto Waffles (Flourless Waffles)

INGREDIENTS

• 2 large eggs

• ½ cup shredded cheddar cheese

Optional Toppings

• ½ tablespoon butter

• ¼ cup whipped cream

• ¼ cup raspberries

• 2 tablespoons Sugar-free maple syrup

INSTRUCTIONS

1. Preheat the waffle maker to medium-high heat.

2. Whisk the eggs in a mixing bowl. Mix the cheese until combined.

3. Pour batter into the waffle maker. Close and cook for 3-5 minutes until done. Repeat, if needed, until all batter is cooked.

4. Serve immediately. Store leftovers in the fridge for 3-5 days.

Bone Broth Latte Recipe for Breakfast in the Morning

INGREDIENTS

- ¾ cup freshly brewed coffee hot

- ½ cup bone broth

- ¼ cup milk dairy or plant-based

- 1 ½ tablespoon Keto sugar substitute or sweetener of choice

- 1 tablespoon butter or coconut oil for dairy-free

- 1 raw egg yolk optional

- 1 tablespoon cacao powder

- ½ teaspoon ground cinnamon

• ¼ teaspoon vanilla extract

INSTRUCTIONS

1. Pour the bone broth into a small saucepan and heat it gently over medium-low heat until it becomes hot and steaming but not boiling.

2. Whisk in the sweetener, butter, optional egg yolk, cacao powder, cinnamon, and vanilla until everything blends well.

3. Pour into your favorite mug, and combine with the coffee.

4. Heat the milk in the small saucepan over medium-low heat until it is warm and steaming but not boiling. Froth the milk using a milk frother or by vigorously whisking it by hand in the saucepan until it becomes frothy.

5. Pour the frothed milk over the hot coffee broth. Garnish with an optional dusting of cinnamon. Serve immediately.

The Best Psyllium Husk Keto Bread

INGREDIENTS

• 6 tablespoons psyllium husk powder

• ¾ cup coconut flour

• 1 ½ teaspoons baking soda

• 1 teaspoon salt

• 8 whole eggs

• ½ cup coconut oil or butter, softened

• ¾ cup hot water

INSTRUCTIONS

1. Preheat oven to 350 °F (175°C).

2. Separate the ingredients by mixing the dry ingredients (psyllium husk powder, coconut flour, baking soda, salt) in a bowl and the wet ingredients (eggs, butter or coconut oil, and hot water) in another bowl.

3. Combine the two bowls together by adding the wet into the dry. Work quickly to mix thoroughly because once the psyllium is activated with water it gels fast! Do not over mix.

4. Transfer to a lightly greased standard 8×4-inch bread loaf pan.

5. Bake for 60 minutes. The best way to tell if the bread is done is to look for a hard and crusty top. It should be dark brown and firm.

6. Remove from the oven and let sit in the bread pan for 15 minutes to settle. Loosen the edges with a knife to release the bread. Cool completely on a wire rack before slicing.

Carnivore Breakfast Muffins (with 5 Keto Variations)

INGREDIENTS

• 9 large eggs

• 8 ounces ground beef

• 1 teaspoon salt

INSTRUCTIONS

1. Preheat the oven to 350 °F (175°C).

2. Lightly grease a standard size muffin tin.

3. Brown the meat in a skillet over medium heat.

4. Whisk eggs in a large bowl. Add meat and salt. Stir to combine.

5. Divide the mixture evenly into the muffin tins. Fill each well ¾ full. Bake for 20 minutes until eggs set.

6. Remove from oven and cool for 5 minutes. Release by running a knife around the edge of each muffin. Pop out and continue cooling on a wire rack or serve. Enjoy leftovers cold or reheat in the oven before serving.

High Protein Strawberry Cheesecake Parfait

INGREDIENTS

• 1/2 cup low-sodium cottage cheese

• 1 tsp vanilla

- 1 tbsp no sugar cheesecake jello pudding (the powder)

- 1/2 cup strawberries

- 1/2 cup non-fat plain Greek yogurt

- 1 tsp honey

INSTRUCTIONS

1. Put all **INGREDIENTS** into mini Cuisinart and blend.

Valentine's Day Protein Packed Parfait

INGREDIENTS

- 4 tart cherries

- 1 tsp vanilla extract

- squirt of lime juice

• 1/2 scoop Vanilla Egg White Protein powder

• 1/2 cup non fat plain Greek yogurt

• 1/2 cup Farmer's Cheese

• mint sprig

• 1/8 cup chopped unsalted Pistachio nuts

INSTRUCTIONS

1. Gather Farmer's cheese, yogurt, protein powder, a squeeze of lime juice, and vanilla and mix in a small Cuisinart or blender.

2. Chop pistachios

3. Put mixed **INGREDIENTS** in a cup and top with cherries, and a tiny bit of lime zest, and chopped pistachios. A sprig of mint will be the surprise hit! Don't skip it!

Copycat Fiber One Muffins

INGREDIENTS

- 1/2 Teaspoon vanilla

- 1 Egg

- 1.5 Cup Fiber One cereal

- 1/2 Cup Swerve brown sugar

- 1/4 Olive oil

- 1 1/3 Cup of Fairlife ultra milk

- Scoop vanilla protein powder

- 1 Cup Bob red mill high fiber oat bran cereal

- 2 teaspoon baking powder

INSTRUCTIONS

1. Preheat oven to 400.

2. Spray the muffin pan with cooking spray so the muffins don't stick.

3. Crush cereal in a baggie with a rolling pin or use a glass like I did. Whatever you have available to crush cereal into a finer consistency.

4. Add milk and vanilla to the cereal and let sit for 5 minutes.

5. In another bowl, beat egg and add in oil.

6. Add the rest of the **INGREDIENTS** (baking powder, protein powder, oat bran, and Swerve brown sugar) to the beaten egg and oil mixture.

7. Add egg mixture to cereal mixture.

8. Fill the muffin pan.

9. Place in oven and bake for 20 minutes. Check at 15 with a toothpick; if it comes out clean, they are done. If not, bake for an additional 5 minutes.

Banana French Toast with Peanut Butter Maple Drizzle

INGREDIENTS

• 1 small banana

• 1 teaspoon cinnamon

• 2 Tablespoon powdered peanut butter

• 1 pat of butter

• Ezekiel bread

• 1/4 cup of skim milk

• 1 whole egg

• 1 Tablespoon sugar-free maple syrup

INSTRUCTIONS

French toast batter.

1. Mix together milk, egg, and cinnamon.

2. Heat a nonstick skillet with a pat of butter.

3. Drench the bread in the batter.

4. When the skillet is hot, put in french toast and cook on each side until brown. About 2 minutes each.

5. While making french toast, make your PB drizzle by following the directions on the PB2 jar. I added more water so that the drizzle could, well, drizzle!

6. When both pieces of toast are nice and brown, put them on the plate and pour on the maple syrup and PB drizzle. Garnish with fruit.

Arugula Egg Goat Cheese Breakfast Wrap

INGREDIENTS

- 1/4 cup tomato, diced

- 1/2 cup arugula

- 1/2 teaspoon coconut oil

- 1 large eggs, beaten

- 1/8 cup goat cheese

- 1 low carb tortilla

INSTRUCTIONS

STEP 1

Warm tortilla in a large skillet over medium heat.

STEP 2

Melt coconut oil in a skillet over medium-high heat.

STEP 3

Add eggs and scramble. Cook for about 2 minutes, sprinkle goat cheese over eggs, add arugula, and continue cooking until cheese is melted.

STEP 4

Add eggs to tortilla and top with diced tomato.

STEP 5

Roll tortilla and enjoy.

Flourless Banana Pancakes

INGREDIENTS

- 1 ripe banana

- 2 large eggs

- 2 tablespoon ground flax meal

- 1/4 teaspoon vanilla

- 1 tablespoon coconut oil

INSTRUCTIONS

1. Mix banana and eggs together in a bowl until smooth. Add ground flaxseed and vanilla extract; mix the batter well.

2. Heat coconut oil in a small skillet over medium-low heat. Scoop batter, about 1/4 cup per pancake, onto the skillet and cook until the center starts to bubble, about 30 seconds. Flip pancakes and cook until bottoms are lightly browned, 1 to 2 minutes more.

Chicken Salad Stuffed Avocado

INGREDIENTS

- 1 tablespoon of cilantro

- 3 ounces chicken (can make own or use rotisserie)

- 3 cherry tomatoes

- 1 tablespoon goat cheese

- 1/2 avocado

INSTRUCTIONS

1. Cut one ripe avocado in half and scoop into bowl. Save the shell as you will use it for serving.

2. Add 3 ounces of cooked chicken (store-bought rotisserie works great!) and mix with avocado.

3. Cut up and mix in three cherry tomatoes.

4. Put mixture back into empty avocado shell.

5. Top it off with goat cheese and cilantro.

LUNCH RECIPES FOR LOW OXALATE DIET

Sweet potato & lentil soup

Ingredients

• 2 tsp medium curry powder

• 3 tbsp olive oil

• 2 onions, grated

• 1 eating apple, peeled, cored and grated

• 3 garlic cloves, crushed

• 20g pack coriander, stalks chopped

• thumb-size piece fresh root ginger, grated

- 800g sweet potatoes

- 1.2l low-sodium vegetable stock

- 100g red lentils

- 300ml milk

- juice 1 lime

Directions

- STEP 1

Put the curry powder into a large saucepan, then toast over a medium heat for 2 mins. Add the olive oil, stirring as the spice sizzles in the pan. Tip in the onions, apple, garlic, coriander stalks and ginger, season, then gently cook for 5 mins, stirring every so often.

- STEP 2

Meanwhile, peel, then grate the sweet potatoes. Tip into the pan with the stock, lentils, milk and seasoning, then simmer, covered, for 20 mins. Blend until smooth using a stick blender. Stir in the lime juice, check the seasoning and serve, topped with roughly-chopped coriander leaves.

Sweet potato & cauliflower lentil bowl

Ingredients

• 1 large sweet potato, skin left on, scrubbed and cut into medium chunks

• 1 cauliflower, cut into large florets, stalk diced

• 1 tbsp garam masala

• 3 tbsp groundnut oil

• 2 garlic cloves

* 200g puy lentils

* thumb-sized piece ginger, grated

* 1 tsp Dijon mustard

* 1½ limes, juiced

* 2 carrots

* ¼ red cabbage

* ½ small pack coriander

Directions

* STEP 1

Heat oven to 200C/180C fan/gas 6. Toss the sweet potato and cauliflower with the garam masala, half the oil and some seasoning. Spread out on a large roasting tray. Add the garlic and roast for 30-35 mins until cooked.

• STEP 2

Meanwhile, put the lentils in a saucepan with 400ml cold water. Bring to the boil, then simmer for 20-25 mins until the lentils are cooked but still have some bite. Drain.

• STEP 3

Remove the garlic cloves from the tray and squish them with the blade of your knife. Put the garlic in a large bowl with the remaining oil, ginger, mustard, a pinch of sugar and one-third of the lime juice. Whisk, then tip in the warm lentils, stir and season to taste. Coarsely grate the carrots, shred the cabbage and roughly chop the coriander. Squeeze over the remaining lime juice and season to taste.

• STEP 4

Divide the lentil mixture between four bowls (or four containers if saving and chilling). Top each serving with a quarter of the carrot slaw and a quarter of the sweet potato and cauliflower mix.

Feta & kale loaded sweet potato

Ingredients

• 2 sweet potatoes

• chickpeas, drained

• 1 red onion, thinly sliced

• 2tbsp red wine vinegar

• 30g feta, cut into small cubes

• 1 tsp caster sugar

• 1tbsp olive oil

• chilli flakes

- 100g kale

- 1tbsp pumpkin seeds, toasted

- rocket

Directions

- STEP 1

Heat oven to 200C/180C fan/gas 6. Prick the sweet potatoes all over with a fork, then put them in a roasting tin and roast for 40 mins. Add the chickpeas to the tray, then roast for 10 mins more, until the potatoes are completely tender and the chickpeas have crisped a little.

- STEP 2

Meanwhile, mix the onion with the vinegar and a pinch of sugar and salt, and set aside to quick pickle. In another bowl, marinate the feta with the oil and chilli flakes.

- STEP 3

When the potatoes are nearly cooked, cook the kale in a pan with 50ml water for 3 mins until wilted, then season to taste. Halve the potatoes, divide between two plates and top each with the kale, chickpeas, red onion (reserving the vinegar), marinated feta and pumpkin seeds. Toss the rocket with the reserved vinegar, then serve on the side.

Red lentil & sweet potato pâté

Ingredicnts

- 1 tbsp olive oil, plus extra for drizzling

- ½ onion, finely chopped

- 1 tsp smoked paprika, plus a little extra

• 1 small sweet potato, peeled and diced

• 140g red lentil

• 3 thyme sprigs, leaves chopped, plus a little extra to decorate (optional)

• 500ml low-sodium vegetable stock (choose a vegan brand, if desired)

• 1 tsp red wine vinegar (choose a vegan brand, if desired)

• pitta bread and vegetable sticks, to serve

Directions

• STEP 1

Heat the oil in a large pan, add the onion and cook slowly until soft and golden. Tip in the paprika and cook for a further 2 mins, then add the sweet potato, lentils, thyme and stock. Bring to a simmer, then cook for 20 mins or until the potato and lentils are tender.

• STEP 2

Add the vinegar and some seasoning, and roughly mash the mixture until you get a texture you like. Chill for 1 hr, then drizzle with olive oil, dust with the extra paprika and sprinkle with thyme sprigs, if you like. Serve with pitta bread and vegetable sticks.

Sweet potato cakes with poached eggs

Ingredients

• 4 eggs

• 50g harissa

• 200g Greek yogurt

• handful micro herbs

For the sweet potato cakes

• 500g sweet potato, peeled and grated

• 200g gluten-free flour

• 1 small pack parsley, chopped

• 4 egg whites

• 50g harissa

• olive oil, for frying

Directions

• STEP 1

To make the potato cakes, squeeze the excess moisture from the sweet potato, then combine with flour, parsley, egg white, harissa and some salt in a bowl until the mixture sticks together. Shape into 8 potato cakes. Heat a little oil in a frying pan. In two batches, fry the potato cakes for 2-3 mins each side or until golden brown and crisp. Keep warm while you repeat with the remaining cakes.

• STEP 2

Poach the eggs in a saucepan of simmering water for 2-3 mins – the yolks should be runny. Remove with a slotted spoon and drain carefully on kitchen paper.

• STEP 3

Spread some harissa in the middle of four serving plates and top with a dollop of yogurt. Add one potato cake to each plate then sandwich another potato cake on top with more yogurt. Top each stack with the remaining yogurt and an egg. Season and drizzle with more harissa and scatter over the micro herbs.

Sweet potato & shallot quesadillas

Ingredients

- 4 small or 2 large sweet potatoes

- 1 tbsp olive oil

- 4 banana shallots, finely sliced into rounds

- 200g frozen broad beans

- 4 corn tortillas

- 60g edam, coarsely grated

Directions

- STEP 1

Prick the potatoes all over with a fork, then put in a microwaveable bowl, cover and microwave on high for 10 mins or until soft in the centre. Meanwhile, heat the oil in a frying pan over a medium heat, add the shallots and cook, stirring often, for 10 mins or until soft and beginning to brown. Remove and set aside.

• STEP 2

Cook the broad beans in a pan of boiling salted water for 3 mins, then drain and run under cold water. Pop half out of their pale thicker skins and leave the rest.

• STEP 3

To assemble, put a tortilla in the same frying pan you used for the shallots, over a medium heat. Scatter over a quarter of the cheese, then squeeze over half the potatoes, skin included, sprinkle over half the onions and broad beans, and finish with another quarter of the cheese. Season well, then put a second tortilla on top.

• STEP 4

Leave to cook and heat through for 2 mins, then flip over to cook the other side for another 2 mins. Tip out onto a board and repeat with the remaining Ingredients. Slice and serve.

Spiced black bean & chicken soup with kale

Ingredients

- 2 tbsp mild olive oil

- 2 fat garlic cloves, crushed

- small bunch coriander stalks finely chopped, leaves picked

- zest 1 lime, then cut into wedges

- 2 tsp ground cumin

- 1 tsp chilli flakes

- 400g can chopped tomatoes

- 400g can black beans, rinsed and drained

- 600ml chicken stock

• 175g kale, thick stalks removed, leaves shredded

• 250g leftover roast or ready-cooked chicken

• 50g feta, crumbled, to serve

• flour & corn tortillas, toasted, to serve

Directions

• STEP 1

Heat the oil in a large saucepan, add the garlic, coriander stalks and lime zest, then fry for 2 mins until fragrant. Stir in the cumin and chilli flakes, fry for 1 min more, then tip in the tomatoes, beans and stock. Bring to the boil, then crush the beans against the bottom of the pan a few times using a potato masher. This will thicken the soup a little.

• STEP 2

Stir the kale into the soup, simmer for 5 mins or until tender, then tear in the chicken and let it heat through. Season to taste with salt, pepper and juice from half the lime, then serve in shallow bowls, scattered with the feta and a few coriander leaves. Serve the remaining lime in wedges for the table, with the toasted tortillas on the side. The longer you leave the chicken in the pan, the thicker the soup will become, so add a splash more stock if you can't serve the soup straight away.

Creamy pesto & kale pasta

Ingredients

- 1 tbsp rapeseed oil

- 2 red onions, thinly sliced

- 300g kale

- 300g wholemeal pasta (penne or mafalda work well)

- 4 tbsp reduced-fat soft cheese

- 4 tbsp fresh or jar pesto, or vegetarian alternative

Directions

- STEP 1

Heat the oil in a large pan over a medium heat. Fry the onions for 10 mins until softened and beginning to caramelise. Add the kale and 100ml water, then cover and cook for 5 mins more, or until the kale has wilted.

- STEP 2

Cook the pasta following pack instructions. Drain, reserving a little of the cooking water. Toss the pasta with the onion mixture, soft cheese and pesto, adding a splash of the reserved cooking water to loosen, if needed. Season.

Curried kale & chickpea soup

Ingredients

* 1 tsp rapeseed or coconut oil

* 1 onion, chopped

* 1 tbsp grated ginger

* 2 garlic cloves, crushed

* 1 sweet potato (about 200g), peeled and cut into 2cm cubes

* 1 tsp turmeric

* 2 tsp ground cumin

* 2 tbsp medium or hot curry powder

* 400g can chickpeas, rinsed

- 150ml low-fat coconut milk

- 500ml vegetable stock (see tip, below)

- 160g kale, chopped

- 1 lime, juiced

- 1 red chilli, finely chopped (optional)

Directions

- STEP 1

Heat the oil in a large pan and fry the onion for 5 mins. Add the ginger and garlic, fry for 1 min more, then stir in the sweet potato, spices and chickpeas. Cook for another 5 mins, adding a little water if the spices stick to the pan.

- STEP 2

Pour in the coconut milk and 400ml of the stock, then bring to a simmer and cook for 8 mins. Season, then transfer a quarter of the soup to a blender and whizz until smooth. Pour in the reserved stock to loosen, if needed, then add back to the pan with the remaining soup. Stir in the kale and cook for 5 mins. Add the lime juice, then ladle into bowls and scatter over the chilli, if you like.

Roast sweet potato & onion tart with goat's cheese

Ingredients

• 3 tbsp olive oil

• 6 medium red onions, finely sliced

• 5 tbsp red wine vinegar

• 100g cranberry sauce

- 1kg sweet potatoes, peeled and cut into small chunks

- 1 tsp chilli flakes

- 2 x 320g sheets ready-rolled puff pastry

- 3 x 100g soft goat's cheese with rind, broken into large chunks

- beaten egg, for glazing

- thyme sprigs, to serve

- a large salad, to serve

Directions

- STEP 1

Heat oven to 200C/180C fan/gas 6. Heat 2 tbsp of the oil in a large non-stick frying pan and cook the onions over a low heat for 20-25 mins or until well softened and lightly browned. Add the vinegar and cranberry sauce, and simmer for 5-10 mins more, stirring until almost all the liquid has disappeared. Leave to cool.

• STEP 2

Meanwhile, put the sweet potatoes in a bowl and toss with the remaining oil, 1/2 tsp salt, 1/2 tsp pepper and the chilli flakes. Arrange on a baking tray and cook for 20 mins, turning halfway, until softened and lightly browned. Leave to cool.

• STEP 3

Reduce oven to 180C/160C fan/gas 4. Line two large baking trays with baking parchment and unroll the pastry sheets on top – trimming the edges neatly at this point will encourage a good rise. Leaving a 2cm gap around the edge, spread the onions over the pastry, then top with the sweet potatoes and goat's cheese. Brush the beaten egg around the border of the pastry and bake in the oven for 35-40 mins or until the pastry is golden and crisp, swapping the shelves after 20 mins.

• STEP 4

Scatter over the thyme, then cut each tart into quarters (or smaller pieces if serving more). Serve with a large leafy salad.

Broccoli and kale green soup

Ingredients

• 500ml stock, made by mixing 1 tbsp bouillon powder and boiling water in a jug

• 1 tbsp sunflower oil

• 2 garlic cloves, sliced

• thumb-sized piece ginger, sliced

• ½ tsp ground coriander

• 3cm/1in piece fresh turmeric root, peeled and grated, or 1/2 tsp ground turmeric

• pinch of pink Himalayan salt

• 200g courgettes, roughly sliced

• 85g broccoli

• 100g kale, chopped

• 1 lime, zested and juiced

• small pack parsley, roughly chopped, reserving a few whole leaves to serve

Directions

• STEP 1

Put the oil in a deep pan, add the garlic, ginger, coriander, turmeric and salt, fry on a medium heat for

2 mins, then add 3 tbsp water to give a bit more moisture to the spices.

• STEP 2

Add the courgettes, making sure you mix well to coat the slices in all the spices, and continue cooking for 3 mins. Add 400ml stock and leave to simmer for 3 mins.

• STEP 3

Add the broccoli, kale and lime juice with the rest of the stock. Leave to cook again for another 3-4 mins until all the vegetables are soft.

• STEP 4

Take off the heat and add the chopped parsley. Pour everything into a blender and blend on high speed until smooth. It will be a beautiful green with bits of dark speckled through (which is the kale). Garnish with lime zest and parsley.

Roasted new potato, kale & feta salad with avocado

Ingredients

• 200g Jersey Royal potatoes, halved

• 2 garlic cloves

• 2 tbsp cold-pressed rapeseed oil

• 1 lemon, juiced

• 1 banana shallot, chopped

• 200g bag kale

• 1 small ripe avocado, flesh scooped out

• ½ tsp Dijon mustard

• 25g feta (or vegetarian alternative), crumbled

• ½-1 tsp chilli flakes

• 1 tbsp pumpkin seeds, toasted

Directions

• STEP 1

Heat oven to 200C/180C fan/gas 6. Boil the potatoes for 10 mins until mostly tender, drain and leave to steam dry. Toss the potatoes in a large roasting tin with the garlic, drizzle over 1 tbsp oil and season. Roast for 20 mins.

• STEP 2

While the potatoes are roasting, squceze half the lemon juice over the shallot and half of the kale, season, then massage gently to encourage the kale to soften.

• STEP 3

Remove the garlic cloves from the oven. Put the rest of the kale on top of the potatoes, drizzle over a little oil, season and return to the oven for 5 mins until crisp.

• STEP 4

Meanwhile, blitz the garlic, avocado, mustard, remaining oil and lemon juice together, add enough water to create a smooth dressing and season to taste. Mix the potatoes and cooked kale into the raw kale salad and tip onto a platter. Drizzle over the dressing, then top with the feta, chilli flakes and pumpkin seeds.

Leek, kale & potato soup topped with shoestring fries

Ingredients

• 4 large potatoes (around 500g), 3 peeled and cubed, 1 left whole with skin on

• 1 tbsp cold pressed rapeseed oil

- 15g butter

- 5 leeks (around 500g), washed and sliced into half moons

- 2 garlic cloves, sliced

- 1 ½l vegetable stock (we used Bouillon)

- 200g kale

- 2 tbsp half-fat crème fraîche

Directions

- STEP 1

Heat oven to 220C/200C fan/ gas 7 and line a baking tray with parchment. Cut the whole potato into matchsticks using a julienne peeler, or shave thin slices using a vegetable peeler, then cut into matchsticks. Pat dry using kitchen paper, then toss with the oil and some seasoning. Spread out on the tray and roast for 15-18 mins.

• STEP 2

Melt the butter in a large saucepan. Add the leeks, chopped potatoes and a pinch of salt, then cook gently for 10 mins until the leeks have softened. Stir in the garlic and cook for 1 min more, then pour in the stock. Simmer for 10-12 mins until the potatoes are soft, then add the kale and cook for 2-3 mins to wilt.

• STEP 3

Stir in the crème fraîche, then blitz with a hand blender and season to taste. Divide the soup between bowls and top with the shoestring fries.

Kale & goat's cheese frittata

Ingredients

- 1 tbsp olive oil

- 2 red onions, thinly sliced

- 200g chopped curly kale

- 2 tbsp balsamic vinegar

- 8 large eggs, lightly beaten with a little seasoning

- 100g firm goat's cheese, broken into chunks

Directions

- STEP 1

Heat oven to 190C/170C fan/gas 5. Heat the oil in a 25cm ovenproof frying pan. Add the onions and cook for 10-15 mins until soft and caramelised. Add the kale and 1 tbsp water, and cook for 5 mins until the kale has wilted. Pour in the balsamic vinegar and bubble for 1 min, then add the eggs. Give everything a quick stir, then leave undisturbed to cook over a low-medium heat for 5 mins until the egg is nearly set and the frittata is turning golden brown on the bottom.

• STEP 2

Scatter the goat's cheese over the top of the frittata. Cook in the oven for 10-15 mins until the cheese is bubbling and the frittata is set in the centre.

Griddled squid, lentil, roast pepper & preserved lemon with tahini

Ingredients

• 3 large red peppers, halved and deseeded

• 4 tbsp extra virgin olive oil, plus a little extra for roasting and frying

• ½ small onion, finely chopped

• 1 celery stick, diced

- 225g puy lentils

- 1 lemon, juiced

- ½ small bunch parsley, chopped

- 600g cleaned and prepared squid

- 2 green and 2 red chillies, halved, deseeded and finely sliced

- 2 garlic cloves, finely sliced

- 1 preserved lemon, flesh removed and discarded, rind very finely sliced

For the tahini dressing

- 4 tbsp tahini

- 2 tbsp Greek yogurt

- 2 tbsp extra virgin olive oil

• 2 garlic cloves, crushed

• ½ lemon, juiced

• ½ small bunch coriander, finely chopped

Directions

• STEP 1

Heat the oven to 200C/180C fan/ gas 6. Put the peppers on a baking tray and brush with some olive oil. Roast for 25-30 mins, until soft and blistered. Leave to cool slightly.

• STEP 2

To make the dressing, combine everything together until it is the consistency of double cream. If it's too thick, add a little water and adjust the seasoning to taste. Set aside. Slice the peppers into strips.

• STEP 3

Heat a little olive oil in a medium pan and fry the onion and celery for 10 mins until soft but not coloured. Tip in the lentils and cover with water. Bring to the boil, then reduce the heat and simmer for 15 mins, or until the lentils are tender, topping up the water if needed.

• STEP 4

Drain the lentils, then spoon into a serving bowl. Season well, then stir in 1 tbsp olive oil, half the lemon juice and the parsley. Leave to cool a bit, then add the peppers.

• STEP 5

Cut the 'wings' from the squid and put them aside with the tentacles. Slice the bodies down one side so they open out, then clean the inside by running a knife blade firmly over the flesh. Score the flesh on the inside, ensuring you don't cut all the way through. Pat dry with kitchen paper, then transfer to a bowl with just enough olive oil to moisten the pieces (about 2 tbsp). Heat a griddle pan until very hot.

• STEP 6

Season the squid and griddle in batches for 20-30 seconds on each side until just golden. Cut into bite-sized pieces, then toss through the lentil salad and drizzle over the remaining lemon juice.

• STEP 7

In a small frying pan, heat 1 tbsp oil and fry the chillies and garlic until golden. Pour over the squid, then toss through the preserved lemon. Serve with the dressing spooned over or on the side.

Sweet & sour radicchio with toasted crumbs & herby lentils

Ingredients

• 5 tbsp extra virgin olive oil or rapeseed oil, plus extra
for drizzling

• 1 small red onion, finely chopped

• 15g flat-leaf parsley, leaves picked and finely chopped,
stalks finely chopped

• 2 garlic cloves, crushed

• 400g can black or green lentils, drained

• 15g mint, leaves picked and finely chopped

• 3 tbsp sherry or red wine vinegar

• 100g sourdough or focaccia, pulsed to fine crumbs in
a food processor

• 1 radicchio (about 500g), quartered, cored and leaves
separated

Directions

• STEP 1

Heat 1 tbsp of the oil in a medium saucepan over a medium heat and fry the onion with a pinch of sea salt flakes for 4-5 mins until starting to soften but not colour.

• STEP 2

Add the parsley stalks and half the garlic to the onions, then tip in the lentils and 300ml water. Bring to a simmer and cook for 5 mins, shuffling the pan occasionally – when ready, the lentils should be loose and a little brothy (but not soupy). Add two-thirds of the chopped parsley leaves, two-thirds of the mint, 1 tbsp more oil and 2 tsp of the vinegar. Simmer for 2 mins, then reduce the heat to low just to keep warm.

• STEP 3

Meanwhile, heat 2 tbsp of the oil in a large frying pan over a medium- high heat. After 45 seconds or so, fry the breadcrumbs for 3-4 mins, tossing to coat and stirring occasionally until golden. Reduce the heat to low, stir in the remaining garlic and parsley leaves, cook for 1 min, then transfer to a bowl. Wipe the pan clean with kitchen paper.

• STEP 4

Heat another 1 tbsp oil in the pan over a medium-high heat and cook the radicchio leaves for 1 min, turning often using tongs until they become glossy and slightly wilted (you may need to do this in batches at first, then put all the leaves in the pan once they've all wilted). Make a gap in the middle using a spoon and add the rest of the vinegar along with 1 tbsp water. Turn off the heat and quickly stir the leaves around the pan to wilt further in the steam. Season with sea salt and the remaining mint.

• STEP 5

Divide the lentils between two shallow bowls or plates. Drizzle with a little more oil, top with the leaves and any pan juices, and scatter over the crumbs to serve.

Veggie shepherd's pie with sweet potato mash

Ingredients

• 1 tbsp olive oil

• 1 large onion, halved and sliced

• 2 large carrots (500g/1lb 2oz in total), cut into sugar-cube size pieces

• 2 tbsp thyme chopped

• 200ml red wine

• 400g can chopped tomatoes

- 2 vegetable stock cubes

- 410g can green lentils

- 950g sweet potatoes, peeled and cut into chunks

- 25g butter

- 85g vegetarian mature cheddar, grated

Directions

- STEP 1

Heat 1 tbsp olive oil in a frying pan, then fry 1 halved and sliced large onion until golden.

- STEP 2

Add 2 large carrots, cut into sugar-cube size pieces and most of the 2 tbsp chopped thyme, reserving a sprinkling for later.

• STEP 3

Pour in 200ml red wine, 150ml water and a 400g chopped tomatoes, then crumble in 2 vegetable stock cubes and simmer for 10 mins.

• STEP 4

Tip in a 410g can green lentils, including the juice, then cover and simmer for another 10 mins until the carrots still have a bit of bite and the lentils are pulpy.

• STEP 5

Meanwhile, boil 950g sweet potatoes, cut into chunks, for 15 mins until tender, drain well, then mash with 25g butter and season to taste.

• STEP 6

Pile the lentil mixture into a pie dish, spoon the mash on top, then sprinkle over 85g grated vegetarian mature cheddar and the remaining thyme. The pie can now be covered and chilled for 2 days, or frozen for up to a month.

• STEP 7

Heat oven to 190C/170C fan/gas 5. Cook for 20 mins if cooking straightaway, or for 40 mins from chilled, until golden and hot all the way through. Serve with broccoli.

Lentil & red pepper salad with a soft egg

Ingredients

• 2 eggs

• 400g can green lentils, rinsed and drained

• 1 small red onion, thinly sliced

• 1 red pepper, finely chopped

• 1 tbsp balsamic vinegar

• handful rocket leaves

• 1 tbsp olive oil

Directions

• STEP 1

Boil the eggs for 6 mins, then quickly cool under cold running water and peel off the shells. Tip the lentils into a bowl with the onion, red pepper and balsamic vinegar. Mix well.

• STEP 2

Put the salad onto a serving dish, then pile the rocket on top. Drizzle with the oil, then halve the eggs and sit them on top of the salad.

Salmon meatballs in spicy lentil gravy

Ingredients

• 2 medium slices white bread

• 450g salmon fillet, cut into rough chucks

• 1 egg white

• 1 tbsp olive oil

For the spicy gravy

• 2 tbsp korma curry paste

• 1 small onion, finely chopped

• 2 red peppers, finely chopped

• 500g carton tomato passata

• 50g red lentils

Directions

• STEP 1

In a food processor, whizz the bread to fine crumbs. Set aside, then whizz the salmon. Add the crumbs and egg white, then pulse to combine. Season. Divide into 12 balls and chill for 30 mins. Can be frozen at this stage for up to 1 month.

• STEP 2

Heat oven to 200C/fan 180C/gas 6. Heat the oil in a non-stick frying pan. Add the fishballs and fry for 1-2 mins until lightly browned. Transfer to a baking tray, bake for 15 mins until golden.

• STEP 3

Wipe the pan, add korma paste and onion, and cook for 5 mins, stirring regularly. Add peppers and cook for 2 mins. Add passata and lentils, bring to the boil, then simmer for 20 mins. Coat fishballs in the gravy and serve.

Coriander roast chicken thighs with puy lentil salad

Ingredients

• 185g puy lentils

• 20g ginger, peeled

• 30g coriander, plus extra leaves to serve

• 1 tsp each garam masala and ground coriander

• ½ tsp ground cumin

• 2 large whole garlic cloves, plus 1 small clove, finely grated

• 2 tbsp lemon juice

• 150g pot plain bio yogurt

• 6 bone-in, skinless chicken thighs

• 1 tbsp fresh turmeric, finely grated

• 1 tbsp rapeseed or olive oil, plus 1 tsp

• 3 red onions (325g), thickly sliced

• 1 large red pepper and 1 large yellow pepper, deseeded and cut into chunks

• 400g cauliflower, cut into small florets

• 1 tsp cumin seeds

Directions

- • STEP 1

Heat the oven to 220C/200C fan/ gas 7. Boil the lentils for 35-40 mins over a medium heat until tender.

- • STEP 2

Meanwhile, put the ginger, fresh coriander, garam masala, the ground coriander, ground cumin and the 2 whole garlic cloves in a large bowl with half the lemon juice and 3 tbsp of the yogurt. Blitz using a hand blender until smooth. Use 4 tbsp of the mixture to coat the chicken thighs in a large bowl. Arrange the chicken on a baking tray in a single layer.

- • STEP 3

Add the remaining yogurt to the remaining spice and herb mixture, along with the turmeric, 1 tsp oil, the grated garlic, 1 tbsp water and remaining lemon juice to taste. Set aside.

• STEP 4

Tip the onions, peppers and cauliflower into the bowl used for the chicken, and toss with 1 tbsp oil to coat in some of the spice mix. Spread the veg out on a baking tray, then put in the oven with the chicken for 30-35 mins until the chicken is cooked through.

• STEP 5

Remove the chicken and wrap in foil to keep it warm. Scatter the cumin seeds over the veg and return to the oven for 5 mins until golden.

• STEP 6

To serve, drain the lentils and put in a serving bowl with the roasted veg and the remaining turmeric yogurt. Gently toss together. Serve with the chicken (taking the meat off the bones), and scatter with the extra coriander

Fennel, cherry & goat's cheese salad with lentils

Ingredients

- 50g walnut halves or pieces

- 250g pack pre-cooked puy lentils

- 1 large fennel bulb, finely sliced, fronds reserved

- 140g cherries, halved and pitted (or small figs, halved)

- 1 tbsp red wine vinegar

- 2 tbsp extra virgin olive oil

- 1 tsp Dijon mustard

- ½ tsp clear honey

• ½ small pack tarragon, roughly chopped

• 100g pack soft goat's cheese (any kind will work, but ash-rolled looks a bit special), thickly sliced and halved

Directions

• STEP 1

Heat a dry frying pan over a low-medium heat. Add the walnuts and cook for 3 mins, stirring frequently, until they smell toasty and the skins are a deep golden brown. Set aside to cool.

• STEP 2

Heat the lentils following pack instructions, then tip into a large bowl and loosen with a fork. Tip the fennel and cherries on top.

• STEP 3

Whisk together the vinegar, oil, mustard, honey and tarragon, then season. Fold the dressing through the lentils, fennel and cherries, then scoop the salad onto a platter. Scatter with the cheese, walnuts and the reserved fennel fronds.

DINNER RECIPES FOR LOW OXALATE DIET

Spiced mushroom & lentil hotpot

Ingredients

- 2 tbsp olive oil

- 1 medium onion, sliced

- 300g mini Portobello mushrooms or chestnut mushrooms, sliced

- 2 garlic cloves, crushed

- 1 ½ tsp ground cumin

- 1 tsp smoked paprika

• 2 x 400g cans green lentils, drained and rinsed (drained weight 240g)

• 1 tbsp soy sauce

• 1 tbsp balsamic vinegar

• 1 medium sweet potato, peeled and very thinly sliced

• 1 large potato, very thinly sliced

• 1 thyme sprig, leaves picked

Directions

• STEP 1

Heat oven to 200C/180C fan/gas 6. Heat half the oil in a medium saucepan. Fry the onion for 3 mins, then add the mushrooms. Cook for another 3 mins, then increase the heat and add the garlic, ground cumin and paprika, and cook for 1 min. Remove from the heat and add the lentils, soy sauce, balsamic vinegar and 100ml water. Season, then tip the mixture into a casserole dish.

• STEP 2

Rinse the saucepan and return to the hob. Add a kettle full of boiled water and bring back to the boil over a high heat. Add the potato slices, cook for 3 mins, then drain. Arrange on top of the lentils, then brush with the remaining oil. Roast in the oven for 25 mins until the potatoes are golden, then scatter over the thyme before serving.

Salad of roast carrots, apple & lentils with chilli & preserved lemons

Ingredients

For the salad

• 350g baby carrots (a mix of colours is best)

- 1½ tbsp extra virgin olive oil

- 250g cooked puy lentils

- 1 red and 1 green chilli, halved, deseeded and very finely sliced

- 2 preserved lemons, rind only, finely sliced, plus 2 tsp brine from the jar

- 1 large or 2 medium tart eating apples

- ½ lemon, juiced

- 10 mint sprigs, leaves torn

- ½ small bunch of coriander, leaves picked

For the dressing

- 2 tbsp white balsamic vinegar

- 6 tbsp extra virgin olive oil

• 1 large garlic clove, finely grated

• 1cm piece of ginger, peeled and finely grated

• ¼ tsp runny honey

Directions

• STEP 1

Heat the oven to 220C/200C fan/gas 7. Trim the carrots, but leave a bit of the tops on. If you can't find baby carrots, halve or quarter larger ones lengthways. Don't peel them, just wash well. Put in a single layer in a roasting tin, add the olive oil, salt and pepper, then toss to coat. Roast for 25-30 mins until tender. Be careful not to overcook.

• STEP 2

Make the dressing by putting the vinegar in a bowl and whisking in all the other Ingredients with a fork.

Season. Put the lentils in a broad shallow serving bowl with half the chilli and a third of the preserved lemon. Season, then toss with about a third of the dressing. Halve and core the apple (there's no need to peel) and cut into matchsticks. Throw into a large mixing bowl with the lemon juice and add the carrots. Add the rest of the preserved lemons and chilli, along with two-thirds of the herbs and the remaining dressing. Scatter the rest of the herbs over the lentils, and put the carrot and apple mixture on top.

Whole baked ricotta with lentils & roasted cherry tomatoes

Ingredients

• 6 banana shallots, quartered

• 90ml olive oil, plus extra for drizzling

• 1 large lemon, zested and juiced

• small pack basil, roughly chopped

• small pack dill, roughly chopped

• 2 x 250g pouches cooked puy lentils

• 150g spinach

• 2 x 250g whole ricotta

• 400g cherry tomatoes on the vine

Directions

• STEP 1

Heat oven to 200C/180C fan/gas 6. Put the shallots in a medium-sized roasting tin, drizzle over 2 tbsp olive oil and season. Roast for 15 mins until golden brown and beginning to soften. Meanwhile, to make a dressing, whisk the remaining olive oil with the lemon zest and juice, stir through half the herbs and season.

- STEP 2

Toss the lentils together with the shallots, spinach and 4 tbsp water. Put the ricotta in the centre of the roasting tin and lay the tomatoes around them. Drizzle the dressing over the lentils and shake the tin a little to combine everything. Drizzle a little olive oil over the ricotta and season everything well. Return to the oven for 30-35 mins or until the ricotta is firm and lightly golden.

- STEP 3

Serve the lentils in shallow bowls topped with spoonfuls of the creamy ricotta and sprinkled with the remaining herbs.

Lentil & lemon fettuccine

Ingredients

- 140g Puy or brown lentils

- 300g dried fettuccine or linguine

- 50g butter

- 1 medium onion, chopped

- 3 garlic cloves, chopped

- zest and juice 1 lemon

- large handful coriander, leaves and stems roughly chopped

- 150g tub Greek yogurt

Directions

- STEP 1

Rinse the lentils in a sieve and place in a medium saucepan. Cover with plenty of water and bring to the boil, then simmer for about 30 mins until tender, adding salt to taste 10 mins into cooking time. Drain thoroughly and keep warm.

• STEP 2

Cook the pasta, then drain and return to the pan. Meanwhile, melt the butter in a frying pan over a medium heat and add the onion. Cook until lightly golden, then add the garlic and cook until fragrant. Stir the lentils, onion and garlic, lemon zest and juice, coriander and yogurt through the cooked pasta. Finish with plenty of freshly ground black pepper and serve on warm plates.

Spiced rice & lentils with cauliflower

Ingredients

• 2 tbsp sunflower oil

• 1 onion, chopped

- 2 carrots, chopped

- 200g basmati rice

- 50g red lentil

- 3 tbsp korma paste

- 1 head cauliflower, cut into florets

- 100g frozen pea

- few toasted cashew nuts, to serve

- natural yogurt, to serve

- mango chutney, to serve

Directions

- STEP 1

Heat the oil in a pan, add the onion and carrots, then fry for 5 mins until lightly coloured. Stir in the rice and lentils, cook for 1 more min, add the curry paste and 900ml water, then bring to the boil. Cover, then simmer for 10 mins.

• STEP 2

Stir in the cauliflower, then cook for 10 mins more until the rice and lentils are tender. Add the peas 2 mins before cooking time is up, stirring through. Top with the nuts, then serve with yogurt and mango chutney in bowls.

Yellow lentil & coconut curry with cauliflower

Ingredients

• 1 tbsp vegetable oil

• 1 onion, thinly sliced

- 2 garlic cloves, crushed

- thumb-sized piece ginger, finely chopped

- 3 tbsp curry paste (we used Bart Veeraswamy Gujurat Masala curry paste)

- 200g yellow lentil, rinsed

- 1 ½l vegetable stock

- 3 tbsp unsweetened desiccated coconut, plus extra to sprinkle if you like

- 1 cauliflower, broken into little florets

- cooked basmati rice and coriander leaves, plus mango chutney and naan bread (optional), to serve

Directions

- STEP 1

Heat the oil in a large saucepan, then add the onion, garlic and ginger. Cook for 5 mins, add the curry paste, then stir-fry for 1 min before adding the lentils, stock and coconut. Bring the mixture to the boil and simmer for 40 mins or until the lentils are soft.

• STEP 2

During the final 10 mins of cooking, stir in the cauliflower to cook. Spoon rice into 4 bowls, top with the curry and sprinkle with coriander leaves, and coconut if you like. Serve with mango chutney and naan bread (optional).

Garlic prawns with puy lentils

Ingredients

• 400g raw, peeled tiger prawn, defrosted if frozen

• 2 red chillies, deseeded and finely chopped

• zest and juice 1 lime

• 2 large garlic cloves, crushed

• 2 tbsp oil

• 200g Puy lentil

For the dressing

• 2 tbsp soy sauce

• 1 tbsp clear honey

• 1 tbsp rice wine vinegar

• 3 tbsp sesame seed, toasted

• bunch coriander, leaves roughly chopped

Directions

• STEP 1

Place the prawns in a shallow dish. Mix together half the finely chopped chilli, lime zest and juice, garlic and oil, then pour over the prawns. Cover and chill for 20 mins to marinate.

• STEP 2

Meanwhile, put the lentils in a pan, cover with twice their depth in water, bring to the boil, then simmer for 15-20 mins until tender. Top up the water if you need to.

• STEP 3

To make the dressing, put the remaining chopped chilli, the soy, honey and vinegar into a small bowl and stir together. Drain the lentils, then tip into a large bowl. Spoon over almost all the dressing while the lentils are hot, tip in the sesame seeds, then mix well.

• STEP 4

Heat a frying pan until really hot. Lift the prawns out of the marinade, then fry for 1-2 mins each side until pink and lightly golden. Pour in the marinade and bring to the boil. Fold the chopped coriander through the lentils, then spoon onto serving plates. Top with the prawns and any pan juices.

Sticky sausage & sweet potato salad

Ingredients

- 8 pork sausages

- 600g sweet potato, cut into thin wedges

- 1 tbsp olive oil

- 2 tbsp wholegrain mustard

- 3 tbsp clear honey

- 200g bag baby spinach

For the dressing

- 5 tbsp olive oil

- 2 tbsp white wine vinegar

- 1 red onion, thinly sliced

Directions

- STEP 1

Heat oven to 200C/180C fan/gas 6. Toss the sausages and potatoes in a roasting tin with the oil. Roast for 30 mins, then mix the mustard and honey together and stir into the tin. Roast for 10 mins more until sticky and cooked.

- STEP 2

Meanwhile, mix together the dressing Ingredients with some seasoning – the onion will soften slightly in the vinegar.

• STEP 3

When the sausages are ready, thickly slice them, then mix back in with the potatoes. Tip the spinach onto plates, pile the sticky sausage slices and potatoes on top, then spoon over the dressing.

Open leek & sweet potato pie

Ingredients

• 3 tbsp olive oil, plus extra for brushing

• 2 large leeks, washed and sliced

• 2 sweet potatoes, peeled and roughly chopped into 2cm cubes

• 1 tsp coriander seeds

• 1 tsp chilli flakes

• 2 fat garlic cloves, crushed

• 150g ricotta

• 2 large eggs

• 1 lemon, zested

• 100g robust leafy greens such as cavalo nero or kale, finely shredded, tough core removed

• 1 small pack dill, chopped

• 1 pack filo pastry (around 12 sheets)

• 80g goat's cheese

• 1 tsp nigella seeds (optional)

• peppery salad, to serve

Directions

- STEP 1

Heat the oil in a large ovenproof frying pan. Add the leeks and a pinch of salt, then cook over a medium heat for a couple of mins until beginning to wilt. Tip in the sweet potato, cover the pan then cook, stirring occasionally, for 15 mins until the potato is mostly softened. Stir in the coriander seeds, chilli flakes, garlic and season. Give everything a gentle stir – you want the potato to remain intact as much as possible – then remove the pan from the heat and set aside to cool slightly.

- STEP 2

In a large bowl, whisk together the ricotta, eggs and lemon zest with some seasoning. Stir in the greens and dill, then scrape in the sweet potato filling, (set aside the frying pan afterwards) and fold everything together. Heat oven to 220C/200C fan/gas 7.

- STEP 3

Lay your first sheet of filo in the frying pan you used for the sweet potato (no need to wash it first). Brush the top with a little oil, then continue to layer the filo, setting each sheet at a different angle and oiling in between the layers until all edges of the pan are covered. Spoon the filling on top of the pastry, dot over the goat's cheese, then crumple the pastry in over the filling, leaving the centre of the pie exposed. Brush the top with a little more oil and scatter over the nigella seeds, if using.

• STEP 4

Turn the hob back on and cook the pie over a medium-low heat for 3 mins to ensure the base is crisp, then transfer to the oven and bake for 12-15 mins until the pastry is crisp and golden. Let the pie cool in the pan for 10 mins before slicing.

Homemade burgers with sweet potato wedges

Ingredients

For the burgers

• 1 tbsp olive oil, plus extra for drizzling

• 1 red onion, finely chopped

• 500g lean minced beef or turkey

• 1 egg

• 12 cream crackers, bashed to fine crumbs

• 2 tsp chilli paste

• 2 tsp garlic paste

• 1 tsp each, tomato ketchup and brown sauce

• 2 tbsp plain flour

• 6 hamburger rolls, toasted, to serve

• toppings of your choice (relish, chutney and salad),
to serve

For the wedges

• 4 sweet potatoes, cut into wedges

• 2 tbsp olive oil

• 1 tsp paprika

Directions

• STEP 1

Heat the oil in a frying pan and fry the onion for about
5 mins or until soft. Leave to cool slightly. When cool,
put the onion in a large bowl with the mince, egg,
bashed crackers, chilli, garlic, ketchup and brown

sauce, and mix well to combine. Divide the mince into 6, roll into balls and flatten each into a nice fat burger.

• STEP 2

Put the flour on a plate, dab each burger to the flour on both sides, then transfer to a baking tray. Wrap with cling film and pop in the fridge for a couple of hours.

• STEP 3

Heat oven to 200C/180C fan/gas 6. To make the wedges, put the sweet potato on a baking tray and drizzle with olive oil. Sprinkle with paprika, season, then give them a good shake or shuffle around with your hands to make sure they're well coated. Roast for 30-40 mins depending on how crisp you like them. Make sure you give them a good shake a couple of times to ensure they cook evenly.

• STEP 4

When the wedges have been cooking for 10 mins, drizzle the burgers with a little olive oil and put them in the oven to cook with the wedges for the remaining 20-30 mins, flipping them halfway. 5 Serve the burgers in the rolls with your choice of toppings, and a good helping of wedges on the side.

Spicy turkey sweet potatoes

Ingredients

• 4 sweet potatoes

• 1 tbsp olive oil

• 1 onion, finely chopped

• 1 garlic clove, crushed

• 500g pack turkey thigh mince

• 500g carton passata

- 3 tbsp barbecue sauce

- ½ tsp cayenne pepper

- 4 tbsp soured cream

- ½ pack chives, finely snipped

Directions

- STEP 1

Heat oven to 200C/180C fan/gas 6. Prick the potatoes, place on a baking tray and bake for 45 mins or until really soft.

- STEP 2

Meanwhile, heat the oil in a frying pan, add the onion and cook gently for 8 mins until softened. Stir in the garlic, then tip in the mince and stir to break up. Cook over a high heat until any liquid has evaporated and the mince is browned, about 10 mins. Pour in the passata, then fill the carton a quarter full of water and tip that in too. Add the barbecue sauce and cayenne, then lower the heat and simmer gently for 15 mins, adding a little extra water if needed. Taste and season.

• STEP 3

When the potatoes are soft, split them down the centre and spoon the mince over the top. Add a dollop of soured cream and a sprinkling of chives

Sweet potato falafels with coleslaw

Ingredients

For the falafels

• 1 large or 2 small sweet potatoes, about 700g/1lb 9oz in total

• 1 tsp ground cumin

- 2 garlic cloves, chopped

- 2 tsp ground coriander

- handful coriander leaves , chopped

- juice ½ lemon

- 100g plain or gram flour

- 1 tbsp olive oil

- 4 wholemeal pitta breads

- 4 tbsp reduced-fat hummus

For the coleslaw

- 2 tbsp red wine vinegar

- 1 tbsp golden caster sugar

- 1 small onion, finely sliced

• 1 medium carrot, grated

• ¼ each white and red cabbage, shredded

Directions

• STEP 1

Heat oven to 200C/180C fan/gas 6. Microwave sweet potato whole for 8-10 mins until tender. Leave to cool a little, then peel. Put the potato, cumin, garlic, ground and fresh coriander, lemon juice and flour into a large bowl. Season, then mash until smooth. Using a tablespoon, shape mix and into 20 balls. Put on an oiled baking sheet, bake for around 15 mins until the bases are golden brown, then flip over and bake for 15 mins more until brown all over.

• STEP 2

Meanwhile, stir the vinegar and sugar together in a large bowl until the sugar has dissolved, toss through the onion, carrot and cabbage, then leave to marinate for 15 mins. To serve, toast the pittas, then split. Fill with salad, a dollop of hummus and the falafels.

Sweet potato, chickpea & chorizo hash

Ingredients

• 600g sweet potatoes, diced

• 1 tbsp sunflower oil

• 1 large red onion, thinly sliced

• 400g cooking chorizo sausages, skinned and crumbled

• 400g can chickpeas, rinsed and drained

• 4 large eggs

• 1 green chilli, thinly sliced into rings

Directions

• STEP 1

Boil the sweet potatoes for 8 mins until tender, then drain. Meanwhile, heat the oil in a large ovenproof pan and cook the onion and chorizo for 5 mins until softened. Add the sweet potatoes and chickpeas and cook for 5 mins more. Roughly break the mixture up with a fork, then flatten it down lightly to form a cake. Cook for a further 8 mins, without stirring, until cooked through, crispy and golden on the bottom.

• STEP 2

Heat grill to high. Break the eggs onto the hash, season, then place the pan under the grill and cook for 2-3 mins until the whites are set. Sprinkle with chilli to serve.

Sweet potato hash, eggs & smashed avo

Ingredients

• 1 large ripe avocado

• 1 lime, juiced

• 1 tbsp olive oil

• 1 red onion, ends trimmed and spiralized on a flat blade

• 2 medium sweet potatoes, ends trimmed and spiralized into thin noodles

• 2 large eggs

• sriracha, for drizzling

Directions

• STEP 1

Smash up the avocado with a fork, leaving some pieces chunky, then add the lime juice and season to taste.

• STEP 2

Heat the oil in a large, non-stick frying pan over a medium heat. Add the onion and cook for 2 mins, then stir in the sweet potato. Season and press the potato into the pan with the back of a wooden spoon. Cook for 10-15 mins, stirring occasionally, until the potato is softened and crisping at the edges.

• STEP 3

Make two spaces in the pan, crack in the eggs and cook for 2-3 mins until the whites are just set and the yolks runny. Dollop on the avocado and drizzle with sriracha to serve.

MAIN COURSE RECIPES FOR LOW OXALATE DIET

One-pot chicken with chorizo & new potatoes

Ingredients

• 1 whole chicken (about 1.5kg), the best quality you can afford

• small knob of butter

• 1 tbsp olive oil

• ½ lemon

• 1 bay leaf

• 1 thyme sprig

• 300g chorizo ring, thickly sliced

• 700g new potatoes, halved (or quartered if really large)

• 12 garlic cloves, left whole and unpeeled

• large splash of dry sherry

• 150ml chicken stock

• handful parsley leaves, roughly chopped

Directions

• STEP 1

Heat oven to 180C/160C fan/gas 4 and season the chicken all over. In a large flameproof casserole dish with a lid, heat the butter and oil until sizzling, then spend a good 15 mins slowly browning the chicken well all over. Remove from the dish and pop the lemon, bay and thyme in the cavity. Set aside.

• STEP 2

Pour most of the oil out of the dish, place back on the heat and sizzle the chorizo for 5 mins until it starts to release its red oil. Throw in the potatoes, sizzle them until they start to colour, then add the garlic. Splash in the sherry, let it bubble down a little, then pour in the stock.

• STEP 3

Nestle the chicken, breast-side up, among the potatoes, place the lid on the dish and cook in the oven for 1 hr 15 mins or until the legs easily come away from the body. Leave the chicken to rest for 10 mins, then scatter with parsley and serve straight from the dish.

Domino potato, cod, prawn & chorizo pie

Ingredients

• 850g floury potatoes, such as Maris Piper

- 500g cod fillet, skin and pin bones removed

- 650ml full-fat milk

- 6 bay leaves

- good pinch of saffron

- 1 tbsp olive oil, plus a drizzle

- 50g butter

- 1 large onion, halved and finely sliced

- 1 fennel, quartered and finely sliced

- 2 garlic cloves, crushed

- 200g chorizo ring, skin removed and sliced

- 50g plain flour

- small bunch parsley, chopped

- 200g king prawns, peeled

- green salad or veg, to serve

Directions

- STEP 1

Peel and thinly slice the potatoes, tip into a pan of cold water and bring to a simmer. Turn off the heat, leave the potatoes in the water for 1 min, then drain and leave to cool in a colander. The potatoes should still feel firm and hold their shape. Put the cod in a wide, deep pan and pour over the milk. Add 2 bay leaves and saffron and bring to a gentle simmer, cover with a lid, then lower the heat and cook for 2 mins. Turn off the heat and leave the fish in the pan to continue cooking for 5 mins more.

- STEP 2

Heat the oil and butter in another large pan, add the onion and fennel and cook for 10 mins until starting to caramelise. Add the garlic and chorizo, stir until the oils are released, then stir in the flour.

• STEP 3

Remove the fish from the milk and set aside the bay leaves. Add the milk to the chorizo pan bit by bit, stirring between additions, until you have a smooth, thick sauce. Stir in the parsley, season and remove from the heat.

• STEP 4

Heat oven to 200C/180C fan/gas 6. Pour half of the sauce into a large casserole dish. Flake the fish into large chunks and scatter over the sauce. Add the prawns and spoon over the rest of the sauce.

• STEP 5

Stack 5-6 potato slices together and trim off the edges to create a rectangle– don't worry if it's not perfect. Continue making stacks of rectangular potatoes until they're all used up. Scatter the trimmings over the sauce, then arrange the slices on top in a domino pattern, fanning them out to cover the surface. Tuck the reserved bay leaves and four others in among the potatoes, season and drizzle with oil. Bake for 45 mins until the potatoes are tender and golden and the sauce is bubbling up around the edges. Serve with green veg or salad.

Warm new potato salad with bacon & blue cheese

Ingredients

• 500g salad potato, halved

• 2 tbsp olive oil

• 2 red onions, each sliced into 6 wedges

• 4 rashers smoked back bacon, trimmed and cut into large pieces

• 140g mushroom, sliced

• 1 tbsp wholegrain mustard

• 1 tbsp red wine vinegar

• 100g bag mixed watercress and spinach salad

• 85g creamy blue cheese (we used St Agur)

Directions

• STEP 1

Heat oven to 220C/fan 200C/gas 7. Place the potatoes in a roasting tin, then rub with 1 tbsp oil and a sprinkling of salt. Roast for 20 mins, then add the onion wedges to the tin, giving everything a good shake. Roast for 20 mins more until the potatoes have turned a deep golden brown and the onions have caramelised and softened. Leave to cool slightly.

• STEP 2

Heat a non-stick frying pan. Dry-fry the bacon until crisp. Add the sliced mushrooms, then fry for 5 mins more until they have softened.

• STEP 3

Meanwhile, make the dressing. Whisk the mustard, vinegar and remaining 1 tbsp oil with a splash of water. Place potatoes, onions, bacon and mushrooms in a large bowl with the salad leaves, pour over the dressing, then toss well. Divide between 4 plates, then crumble over the blue cheese.

Warm new potato & smoked mackerel salad

Ingredients

• 350g new potato

• 100g crème fraîche

• 1 tsp horseradish cream

• juice of 1 lemon

• 2 smoked mackerel fillets (about 200g/8oz total weight), skinned and flaked

• 85g bag watercress

Directions

• STEP 1

Cook the potatoes in a large pan of boiling salted water for 15-20 minutes or until tender.

• STEP 2

While the potatoes are cooking, mix the crème fraîche in a large bowl with the horseradish cream and lemon juice. Season well with freshly ground black pepper (there's no need for salt because of the saltiness of the smoked mackerel).

• STEP 3

Drain the potatoes, halve and set aside to cool down for a few minutes. Tip into the crème fraîche mix and stir so it coats them and becomes quite runny. Now add the smoked mackerel and watercress and toss gently together. Pile on two plates and serve straight away (it's best while still warm).

Curried chicken & new potato traybake

Ingredients

• 8 chicken drumsticks

• 3 tbsp olive oil

- 1 tsp garlic paste

- 1 tsp ginger paste

- 1 tsp garam masala

- 1 tsp turmeric

- 150ml pot natural yogurt

- 500g new potatoes, halved

- 4 large tomatoes, roughly chopped

- 1 red onion, finely chopped

- small pack coriander, roughly chopped

Directions

- STEP 1

Put the drumsticks in a large bowl with 1 tbsp oil, the garlic, ginger, garam masala, turmeric and 2 tbsp yogurt. Toss together with your hands until coated. Leave to marinate for at least 30 mins (can be left in the fridge overnight). Heat oven to 180C/160C fan/gas 4.

• STEP 2

Put the potatoes in a large roasting tin with the remaining oil and plenty of seasoning. Add the chicken drumsticks and bake for 40-45 mins until cooked and golden.

• STEP 3

Scatter the tomatoes, onion, coriander and some seasoning over the chicken and potatoes, with the remaining yogurt served on the side.

Vegan chickpea curry jacket potatoes

Ingredients

- 4 sweet potatoes

- 1 tbsp coconut oil

- 1 ½ tsp cumin seeds

- 1 large onion, diced

- 2 garlic cloves, crushed

- thumb-sized piece ginger, finely grated

- 1 green chilli, finely chopped

- 1 tsp garam masala

- 1 tsp ground coriander

* ½ tsp turmeric

* 2 tbsp tikka masala paste

* 2 x 400g can chopped tomatoes

* 2 x 400g can chickpeas, drained

* lemon wedges and coriander leaves, to serve

Directions

* STEP 1

Heat oven to 200C/180C fan/gas 6. Prick the sweet potatoes all over with a fork, then put on a baking tray and roast in the oven for 45 mins or until tender when pierced with a knife.

* STEP 2

Meanwhile, melt the coconut oil in a large saucepan over medium heat. Add the cumin seeds and fry for 1 min until fragrant, then add the onion and fry for 7-10 mins until softened.

• STEP 3

Put the garlic, ginger and green chilli into the pan, and cook for 2-3 mins. Add the spices and tikka masala paste and cook for a further 2 mins until fragrant, then tip in the tomatoes. Bring to a simmer, then tip in the chickpeas and cook for a further 20 mins until thickened. Season.

• STEP 4

Put the roasted sweet potatoes on four plates and cut open lengthways. Spoon over the chickpea curry and squeeze over the lemon wedges. Season, then scatter with coriander before serving.

Miso chilli steak with crispy sweet potatoes

Ingredients

- 2 large sweet potatoes, cut into wedges

- 1 tbsp vegetable oil, plus a little extra

- 1 tbsp sesame seed

- 1 tbsp miso paste

- juice 1 lemon

- 1 tbsp hot chilli sauce (sriracha is nice)

- 1 tbsp mirin

- 2 bavette or other lean steaks (about 200g each)

- large handful watercress leaves, to serve

Directions

- STEP 1

Heat oven to 200C/180C fan/gas 6. Put the potato wedges on a baking tray and rub with the oil. Sprinkle the sesame seeds and some seasoning over. Bake for 25 mins or until crisp at the edges.

• STEP 2

In a small bowl, mix together the miso, lemon juice, chilli sauce and mirin. Rub the steaks with a tiny bit of oil and some seasoning. Spoon 1 tbsp of the sauce over each steak and rub into both sides.

• STEP 3

Heat a griddle pan until really hot, cook the steaks for 2 mins each side, or longer if you prefer it well done. Brush more of the sauce over after you turn them. Transfer to a plate, cover loosely with foil, and leave to rest for 5 mins. Serve the steaks sliced, with extra sauce, the potatoes and watercress.

Sausage, kale & gnocchi one-pot

Ingredients

- 1 tbsp olive oil

- 6 pork sausages

- 1 tsp chilli flakes

- 1 tsp fennel seeds (optional)

- 500g fresh gnocchi

- 500ml chicken stock (fresh if you can get it)

- 100g chopped kale

- 40g parmesan, finely grated

Directions

• STEP 1

Heat the oil in a large high-sided frying pan over a medium heat. Squeeze the sausages straight from their skins into the pan, then use the back of a wooden spoon to break the meat up. Sprinkle in the chilli flakes and fennel seeds, if using, then fry until the sausagemeat is crisp around the edges. Remove from the pan with a slotted spoon.

• STEP 2

Tip the gnocchi into the pan, fry for a minute or so, then pour in the chicken stock. Once bubbling, cover the pan with a lid and cook for 3 mins, then stir in the kale. Cook for 2 mins more or until the gnocchi is tender and the kale has wilted. Stir in the parmesan, then season with black pepper and scatter the crisp sausagemeat over the top.

Red lentil, chickpea & chilli soup

Ingredients

- 2 tsp cumin seeds

- large pinch chilli flakes

- 1 tbsp olive oil

- 1 red onion, chopped

- 140g red split lentils

- 850ml vegetable stock or water

- 400g can tomatoes, whole or chopped

- 200g can chickpeas or ½ a can, drained and rinsed (freeze leftovers)

• small bunch coriander, roughly chopped (save a few leaves, to serve)

• 4 tbsp 0% Greek yogurt, to serve

Directions

• STEP 1

Heat a large saucepan and dry-fry 2 tsp cumin seeds and a large pinch of chilli flakes for 1 min, or until they start to jump around the pan and release their aromas.

• STEP 2

Add 1 tbsp olive oil and 1 chopped red onion, and cook for 5 mins.

• STEP 3

Stir in 140g red split lentils, 850ml vegetable stock or water and a 400g can tomatoes, then bring to the boil. Simmer for 15 mins until the lentils have softened.

• STEP 4

Whizz the soup with a stick blender or in a food processor until it is a rough purée, pour back into the pan and add a 200g can drained and rinsed chickpeas.

• STEP 5

Heat gently, season well and stir in a small bunch of chopped coriander, reserving a few leaves to serve. Finish with 4 tbsp 0% Greek yogurt and extra coriander leaves.

Coconut & kale fish curry

Ingredients

• 1 tbsp rapeseed oil

• 1 onion, sliced

• thumb-sized piece ginger, sliced into matchsticks

- 1 tsp turmeric

- 3-4 tbsp mild curry paste (Keralan works well)

- 150g cherry tomatoes, halved

- 150g kale, chopped

- 1 red chilli, halved

- 325ml reduced fat coconut milk

- 300ml low-salt stock

- 250g brown rice

- 100g frozen king prawns

- 2 cod fillets, cut into chunks

- 2 limes, juiced

- ½ small bunch coriander, chopped

• handful of toasted coconut flakes (optional)

Directions

• STEP 1

Heat the oil in a casserole dish. Cook the onion with a pinch of salt for 10 mins until it starts to caramalise. Stir through the ginger, turmeric and curry paste, and cook for 2 mins.

• STEP 2

Add the tomatoes, kale and chilli, and pour in the coconut milk and stock. Simmer for 10-15 mins or until the tomatoes begin to soften. Scoop out the chilli and discard.

• STEP 3

Cook the rice following pack instructions. Gently stir the prawns and cod through the curry, then cook for another 3-5 mins. Squeeze over the lime and stir through half of the coriander. To serve, scatter over the remaining coriander and the coconut flakes, if you like. Serve with the rice.

Veggie tahini lentils

Ingredients

• 50g tahini

• zest and juice 1 lemon

• 2 tbsp olive oil

• 1 red onion, thinly sliced

• 1 garlic clove, crushed

• 1 yellow pepper, thinly sliced

• 200g green beans, trimmed and halved

• 1 courgette, sliced into half moons

• 100g shredded kale

• 250g pack pre-cooked puy lentils

Directions

• STEP 1

In a jug, mix the tahini with the zest and juice of the lemon and 50ml of cold water to make a runny dressing. Season to taste, then set aside.

• STEP 2

Heat the oil in a wok or large frying pan over a medium-high heat. Add the red onion, along with a pinch of salt, and fry for 2 mins until starting to soften and colour. Add the garlic, pepper, green beans and courgette and fry for 5 min, stirring frequently.

• STEP 3

Tip in the kale, lentils and the tahini dressing. Keep the pan on the heat for a couple of mins, stirring everything together until the kale is wilted and it's all coated in the creamy dressing.

Kale with chana & coconut

Ingredients

- 1 tbsp butter

- 1 onion, finely chopped

- thumb-sized piece ginger, grated

- 2 heaped tsp cumin seeds

- 1 tsp turmeric

- 1 tsp ground coriander

- 2 tbsp tomato purée

• 200g kale, large stalks removed, leaves finely shredded

• 400g can chickpeas, drained

• 250ml vegetable stock

• 50g fresh coconut, grated

• 4 heaped tbsp Greek-style yogurt

• 1 tbsp mango chutney

To serve

• 1 tbsp vegetable oil

• 3 garlic cloves, thinly sliced

• 2 tbsp freeze-dried curry leaves (optional)

Directions

- STEP 1

Heat the butter in a deep frying pan, add the onion, then soften gently for 5 mins. Turn up the heat and add the ginger and spices; fry for 2 mins until fragrant. Stir in the tomato purée.

- STEP 2

Add the kale, chickpeas, stock and two-thirds of the coconut, stir well, then cover the pan. Bring to a simmer and let the kale steam for 10 mins until very well wilted. Mix in the yogurt and chutney, then season to taste - don't boil once the yogurt has gone in. Remove the pan from the heat, and leave it covered to stay warm.

- STEP 3

Heat the oil in a small saucepan. When it's hot, add the garlic (and curry leaves, if using) and sizzle for 30 secs-1 min until the garlic begins to turn golden. Spoon the oil, garlic and curry leaves over the chickpeas and kale, then finish with the remaining coconut.

Prosciutto, kale & butter bean stew

Ingredients

• 80g pack prosciutto, torn into pieces

• 2 tbsp olive oil

• 1 fennel bulb, sliced

• 2 garlic clove, crushed

• 1 tsp chilli flakes

• 4 thyme sprigs

• 150ml white wine or chicken stock

• 2 x 400g cans butter beans

• 400g can cherry tomatoes

• 200g bag sliced kale

Directions

• STEP 1

Fry the prosciutto in a dry saucepan over a high heat until crisp, then remove half with a slotted spoon and set aside. Turn the heat down to low, pour in the oil and tip in the fennel with a pinch of salt. Cook for 5 mins until softened, then throw in the garlic, chilli flakes and thyme and cook for a further 2 mins, then pour in the wine or stock and bring to a simmer.

• STEP 2

Tip both cans of butter beans into the stew, along with their liquid, then add the tomatoes, season well and bring everything to a simmer. Cook, undisturbed, for 5 mins, then stir through the kale. Once wilted, ladle the stew into bowls, removing the thyme sprigs and topping each portion with the remaining prosciutto.

Kale pesto

Ingredients

• 85g pine nut, toasted

• 85g parmesan (or vegetarian alternative), coarsely grated, plus extra to serve (optional)

• 3 garlic cloves

• 75ml extra-virgin olive oil, plus extra to serve

• 75ml olive oil

• 85g kale

• juice 1 lemon

• spaghetti or linguine, to serve

Directions

• STEP 1

Put the pine nuts, Parmesan, garlic, oils, kale and lemon juice in a food processor and whizz to a paste. Season to taste. Stir through hot pasta to serve, topping with extra Parmesan and olive oil, if you like.

• STEP 2

To store, put in a container or jar, cover the surface with a little more olive oil and keep in the fridge for a week, or freeze for up to a month.

SECTION V: FINALLY!

In order to diagnose kidney stones, your physician will ask for a medical history, will most likely do a physical exam and imaging testing, and urine and blood tests. Image testing is done so your physician can know the exact shape and size of the stone. It can be done with high resolution CT scan, KUB x-ray or intravenous pyelogram.

The healthcare provider may also request a collection of 24-hour urine to test for levels of stone-forming minerals and stone-preventing substances. A blood test can check for calcium, phosphorus, and uric acid levels. In addition, a stone analysis is performed if a stone comes out of your body in order to determine the cause and plan to prevent it from happening again.

You healthcare provider will determine how often to collect urine samples in order to check how well limiting the amount of oxalate in your food is working.

Long-term Maintenance and Sustainability

To stick with a low oxalate diet for the long haul, it's all about staying informed, planning ahead, and keeping an eye on what you eat. Here are some tips to make it easier:

1. Know Your Foods: Get familiar with which foods are high and low in oxalates. Keep a handy list so you can easily pick out the right foods when you're shopping or cooking.

2. Plan Your Meals: Take some time to plan your meals ahead of schedule. This helps you avoid grabbing high oxalate foods on a whim.

3. Keep it Balanced: Even though you're cutting down on oxalates, make sure your diet stays balanced and nutritious. Mix up your fruits, veggies, proteins, and grains wisely.

4. Read Labels: Get into the habit of checking food labels for oxalate content, especially for packaged foods and sauces.

5. Cooking Tips: Certain cooking methods can lower oxalate levels in foods. For example, boiling veggies can reduce oxalates more than steaming or microwaving.

6. Watch Supplements: Some supplements and medications can contain oxalates. Talk to your healthcare provider about alternatives if needed.

7. Stay Hydrated: Drinking enough water is crucial—it helps prevent kidney stones often linked to high oxalate levels in urine.

8. Monitor and Adjust: Pay attention to how your body reacts to your diet. Adjust your food choices as needed based on how you feel.

9. Get Support: Don't hesitate to reach out to healthcare pros, dietitians, or online communities for advice and encouragement.

10. Commit Long-term: Remember, sticking to a low oxalate diet is a marathon, not a sprint. It might take time to figure out what works best for you, but consistency pays off.

By following these tips, you can manage a low oxalate diet over time, supporting your overall health and well-being along the way.

www.ingramcontent.com/pod-product-compliance
Lightning Source LLC
Chambersburg PA
CBHW070656250726
48662CB00001B/156